MW00878993

This book belongs to:

_____

📓 DATE		# WEEK

🔖 NAME	🧪 DOSAGE	🕐 TIME
		: AM / PM
		: AM / PM
		: AM / PM
		: AM / PM
		: AM / PM
		: AM / PM
		: AM / PM
		: AM / PM
		: AM / PM
		: AM / PM
		: AM / PM
		: AM / PM
		: AM / PM
		: AM / PM
		: AM / PM

🫁 SIDE EFFECTS	📝 ADDITIONAL NOTES

PHYSICAL CONDITION

☀️ SLEEP	⬜⬜⬜⬜⬜	🥛 WATER	⬜⬜⬜⬜⬜
⚡ ENERGY	⬜⬜⬜⬜⬜	🏃 ACTIVITY	⬜⬜⬜⬜⬜

🗓 DATE		# WEEK

💊 NAME	🌱 DOSAGE	⏱ TIME	
		:	AM / P
		:	AM / P
		:	AM / P
		:	AM / P
		:	AM / P
		:	AM / P
		:	AM / P
		:	AM / P
		:	AM / P
		:	AM / P
		:	AM / P
		:	AM / P
		:	AM / P
		:	AM / P
		:	AM / P

🧠 SIDE EFFECTS	📝 ADDITIONAL NOTES
•	
•	
•	
•	
•	

PHYSICAL CONDITION	
🌙 SLEEP	🥤 WATER
⚡ ENERGY	🏃 ACTIVITY

| 🗓 DATE | | # WEEK | |

🖊 NAME	🌱 DOSAGE	⏰ TIME	
		:	AM / PM
		:	AM / PM
		:	AM / PM
		:	AM / PM
		:	AM / PM
		:	AM / PM
		:	AM / PM
		:	AM / PM
		:	AM / PM
		:	AM / PM
		:	AM / PM
		:	AM / PM
		:	AM / PM
		:	AM / PM
		:	AM / PM

🗣 SIDE EFFECTS	📝 ADDITIONAL NOTES

PHYSICAL CONDITION

🌙 SLEEP	▭▭▭▭▭	🥛 WATER	▭▭▭▭▭
⚡ ENERGY	▭▭▭▭▭	🏃 ACTIVITY	▭▭▭▭▭

📅 DATE		# WEEK	

💊 NAME	🌿 DOSAGE	⏱ TIME	
		:	AM / P
		:	AM / P
		:	AM / P
		:	AM / P
		:	AM / P
		:	AM / P
		:	AM / P
		:	AM / P
		:	AM / P
		:	AM / P
		:	AM / P
		:	AM / P
		:	AM / P
		:	AM / P
		:	AM / P

🧠 SIDE EFFECTS	📝 ADDITIONAL NOTES
•	
•	
•	
•	
•	

PHYSICAL CONDITION	
🌙 SLEEP	🥛 WATER
☀ ENERGY	🏃 ACTIVITY

DATE	# WEEK

NAME	🌱 DOSAGE	⏰ TIME
		: AM / PM
		: AM / PM
		: AM / PM
		: AM / PM
		: AM / PM
		: AM / PM
		: AM / PM
		: AM / PM
		: AM / PM
		: AM / PM
		: AM / PM
		: AM / PM
		: AM / PM
		: AM / PM
		: AM / PM

SIDE EFFECTS	📝 ADDITIONAL NOTES

PHYSICAL CONDITION

SLEEP	⬭⬭⬭⬭⬭	🥛 WATER	⬭⬭⬭⬭⬭
ENERGY	⬭⬭⬭⬭⬭	🏃 ACTIVITY	⬭⬭⬭⬭⬭

📅 DATE		# WEEK	

💊 NAME	🌱 DOSAGE	⏰ TIME	
		:	AM
		:	AM
		:	AM
		:	AM
		:	AM
		:	AM
		:	AM
		:	AM
		:	AM
		:	AM
		:	AM
		:	AM
		:	AM
		:	AM
		:	AM

🗣 SIDE EFFECTS	📝 ADDITIONAL NOTES
·	
·	
·	
·	
·	

PHYSICAL CONDITION	
🌙 SLEEP	🥤 WATER
⚡ ENERGY	🏃 ACTIVITY

DATE		# WEEK

NAME	DOSAGE	TIME	
		:	AM / PM
		:	AM / PM
		:	AM / PM
		:	AM / PM
		:	AM / PM
		:	AM / PM
		:	AM / PM
		:	AM / PM
		:	AM / PM
		:	AM / PM
		:	AM / PM
		:	AM / PM
		:	AM / PM
		:	AM / PM
		:	AM / PM

SIDE EFFECTS	ADDITIONAL NOTES

PHYSICAL CONDITION

SLEEP		WATER	
ENERGY		ACTIVITY	

📅 DATE		# WEEK	

💊 NAME	🌱 DOSAGE	🕐 TIME	
		:	AM / P
		:	AM / P
		:	AM / P
		:	AM / P
		:	AM / P
		:	AM / P
		:	AM / P
		:	AM / P
		:	AM / P
		:	AM / P
		:	AM / P
		:	AM / P
		:	AM / P
		:	AM / P
		:	AM / P

🗣 SIDE EFFECTS	📝 ADDITIONAL NOTES
•	
•	
•	
•	
•	

PHYSICAL CONDITION	
🌙 SLEEP	🥤 WATER
⚡ ENERGY	🏃 ACTIVITY

📅 DATE		#️⃣ WEEK	

💊 NAME	🪴 DOSAGE	💊 TIME	
		:	AM / PM
		:	AM / PM
		:	AM / PM
		:	AM / PM
		:	AM / PM
		:	AM / PM
		:	AM / PM
		:	AM / PM
		:	AM / PM
		:	AM / PM
		:	AM / PM
		:	AM / PM
		:	AM / PM
		:	AM / PM
		:	AM / PM

🦠 SIDE EFFECTS	📝 ADDITIONAL NOTES

PHYSICAL CONDITION			
💤 SLEEP	⬜⬜⬜⬜⬜	🥤 WATER	⬜⬜⬜⬜⬜
⚡ ENERGY	⬜⬜⬜⬜⬜	🏃 ACTIVITY	⬜⬜⬜⬜⬜

📅 DATE		# WEEK

💊 NAME	🌿 DOSAGE	🕐 TIME
		: AM / P
		: AM / P
		: AM / P
		: AM / P
		: AM / P
		: AM / P
		: AM / P
		: AM / P
		: AM / P
		: AM / P
		: AM / P
		: AM / P
		: AM / P
		: AM / P
		: AM / P

🧠 SIDE EFFECTS	📝 ADDITIONAL NOTES
•	
•	
•	
•	
•	

PHYSICAL CONDITION	
🌙 SLEEP	🥛 WATER
☀️ ENERGY	🏃 ACTIVITY

DATE		# WEEK	

NAME	🌱 DOSAGE	🕐 TIME	
		:	AM / PM
		:	AM / PM
		:	AM / PM
		:	AM / PM
		:	AM / PM
		:	AM / PM
		:	AM / PM
		:	AM / PM
		:	AM / PM
		:	AM / PM
		:	AM / PM
		:	AM / PM
		:	AM / PM
		:	AM / PM
		:	AM / PM

SIDE EFFECTS	📝 ADDITIONAL NOTES

PHYSICAL CONDITION	
SLEEP	🥛 WATER
ENERGY	🏃 ACTIVITY

📅 DATE		# WEEK

💊 NAME	🌱 DOSAGE	⏰ TIME
		: AM
		: AM
		: AM
		: AM
		: AM
		: AM
		: AM
		: AM
		: AM
		: AM
		: AM
		: AM
		: AM
		: AM
		: AM

🤕 SIDE EFFECTS

-
-
-
-
-

📝 ADDITIONAL NOTES

PHYSICAL CONDITION

🌙 SLEEP		🥤 WATER	
⚡ ENERGY		🏃 ACTIVITY	

DATE	# WEEK

NAME	DOSAGE	TIME
		: AM / PM
		: AM / PM
		: AM / PM
		: AM / PM
		: AM / PM
		: AM / PM
		: AM / PM
		: AM / PM
		: AM / PM
		: AM / PM
		: AM / PM
		: AM / PM
		: AM / PM
		: AM / PM
		: AM / PM
		: AM / PM

SIDE EFFECTS	ADDITIONAL NOTES

PHYSICAL CONDITION

SLEEP		WATER	
ENERGY		ACTIVITY	

📅 DATE		# WEEK

💊 NAME	🌱 DOSAGE	⏰ TIME
		: AM / P
		: AM / P
		: AM / P
		: AM / P
		: AM / P
		: AM / P
		: AM / P
		: AM / P
		: AM / P
		: AM / P
		: AM / P
		: AM / P
		: AM / P
		: AM / P
		: AM / P

🧠 SIDE EFFECTS	📝 ADDITIONAL NOTES
•	
•	
•	
•	
•	

PHYSICAL CONDITION	
🌙 SLEEP	💧 WATER
☀️ ENERGY	🏃 ACTIVITY

DATE	# WEEK

NAME	DOSAGE	TIME
		: AM / PM
		: AM / PM
		: AM / PM
		: AM / PM
		: AM / PM
		: AM / PM
		: AM / PM
		: AM / PM
		: AM / PM
		: AM / PM
		: AM / PM
		: AM / PM
		: AM / PM
		: AM / PM
		: AM / PM
		: AM / PM

SIDE EFFECTS	ADDITIONAL NOTES

PHYSICAL CONDITION		
SLEEP	WATER	
ENERGY	ACTIVITY	

📅 DATE			# WEEK	

💊 NAME	🌱 DOSAGE	🕐 TIME	
		:	AM / P
		:	AM / P
		:	AM / P
		:	AM / P
		:	AM / P
		:	AM / P
		:	AM / P
		:	AM / P
		:	AM / P
		:	AM / P
		:	AM / P
		:	AM / P
		:	AM / P
		:	AM / P
		:	AM / P

🧠 SIDE EFFECTS	📝 ADDITIONAL NOTES
•	
•	
•	
•	
•	

PHYSICAL CONDITION	
🌙 SLEEP	💧 WATER
⚡ ENERGY	🏃 ACTIVITY

DATE		# WEEK

NAME	🪴 DOSAGE	💊 TIME
		: AM / PM
		: AM / PM
		: AM / PM
		: AM / PM
		: AM / PM
		: AM / PM
		: AM / PM
		: AM / PM
		: AM / PM
		: AM / PM
		: AM / PM
		: AM / PM
		: AM / PM
		: AM / PM
		: AM / PM
		: AM / PM

SIDE EFFECTS	📝 ADDITIONAL NOTES

PHYSICAL CONDITION	
SLEEP	🥛 WATER
ENERGY	🏃 ACTIVITY

📅 DATE		#️⃣ WEEK

💊 NAME	🌱 DOSAGE	🕐 TIME
		: AM
		: AM
		: AM
		: AM
		: AM
		: AM
		: AM
		: AM
		: AM
		: AM
		: AM
		: AM
		: AM
		: AM
		: AM

🗣 SIDE EFFECTS	📝 ADDITIONAL NOTES
•	
•	
•	
•	
•	

PHYSICAL CONDITION	
🌙 SLEEP	🥛 WATER
☀ ENERGY	🏃 ACTIVITY

📅 DATE		# WEEK

🔖 NAME	🏺 DOSAGE	🕐 TIME
		: AM / PM
		: AM / PM
		: AM / PM
		: AM / PM
		: AM / PM
		: AM / PM
		: AM / PM
		: AM / PM
		: AM / PM
		: AM / PM
		: AM / PM
		: AM / PM
		: AM / PM
		: AM / PM
		: AM / PM
		: AM / PM

🦴 SIDE EFFECTS	📝 ADDITIONAL NOTES

PHYSICAL CONDITION	
💤 SLEEP ☐☐☐☐☐	🥛 WATER ☐☐☐☐☐
⚡ ENERGY ☐☐☐☐☐	🏃 ACTIVITY ☐☐☐☐☐

📅 DATE		# WEEK	

💊 NAME	🌱 DOSAGE	⏰ TIME	
		:	AM /
		:	AM /
		:	AM /
		:	AM /
		:	AM /
		:	AM /
		:	AM /
		:	AM /
		:	AM /
		:	AM /
		:	AM /
		:	AM /
		:	AM /
		:	AM /
		:	AM /

🧠 SIDE EFFECTS	📝 ADDITIONAL NOTES
•	
•	
•	
•	
•	

PHYSICAL CONDITION			
🌙 SLEEP	⬭⬭⬭⬭⬭	🥛 WATER	⬭⬭⬭⬭⬭
☀️ ENERGY	⬭⬭⬭⬭⬭	🏃 ACTIVITY	⬭⬭⬭⬭⬭

▦ DATE		# WEEK

✎ NAME	🌱 DOSAGE	⏱ TIME
		: AM / PM
		: AM / PM
		: AM / PM
		: AM / PM
		: AM / PM
		: AM / PM
		: AM / PM
		: AM / PM
		: AM / PM
		: AM / PM
		: AM / PM
		: AM / PM
		: AM / PM
		: AM / PM
		: AM / PM
		: AM / PM

🖐 SIDE EFFECTS

📝 ADDITIONAL NOTES

PHYSICAL CONDITION

☽ SLEEP		🥛 WATER	
☀ ENERGY		🏃 ACTIVITY	

📅 DATE		# WEEK

💊 NAME	🌱 DOSAGE	🕐 TIME	
		:	AM / PM
		:	AM / PM
		:	AM / PM
		:	AM / PM
		:	AM / PM
		:	AM / PM
		:	AM / PM
		:	AM / PM
		:	AM / PM
		:	AM / PM
		:	AM / PM
		:	AM / PM
		:	AM / PM
		:	AM / PM
		:	AM / PM

🧠 SIDE EFFECTS	📝 ADDITIONAL NOTES
•	
•	
•	
•	
•	

PHYSICAL CONDITION	
🌙 SLEEP	💧 WATER
⚡ ENERGY	🏃 ACTIVITY

DATE		# WEEK	

NAME	DOSAGE	TIME	
		:	AM / PM
		:	AM / PM
		:	AM / PM
		:	AM / PM
		:	AM / PM
		:	AM / PM
		:	AM / PM
		:	AM / PM
		:	AM / PM
		:	AM / PM
		:	AM / PM
		:	AM / PM
		:	AM / PM
		:	AM / PM
		:	AM / PM

SIDE EFFECTS	ADDITIONAL NOTES

PHYSICAL CONDITION

SLEEP	⬡⬡⬡⬡⬡	WATER	⬡⬡⬡⬡⬡
ENERGY	⬡⬡⬡⬡⬡	ACTIVITY	⬡⬡⬡⬡⬡

📅 DATE		# WEEK

💊 NAME	🌱 DOSAGE	🕐 TIME
		: AM
		: AM
		: AM
		: AM
		: AM
		: AM
		: AM
		: AM
		: AM
		: AM
		: AM
		: AM
		: AM
		: AM
		: AM

🧠 SIDE EFFECTS	📝 ADDITIONAL NOTES
•	
•	
•	
•	
•	

PHYSICAL CONDITION	
🌙 SLEEP	💧 WATER
⚡ ENERGY	🏃 ACTIVITY

DATE	# WEEK

NAME	DOSAGE	TIME
		: AM / PM
		: AM / PM
		: AM / PM
		: AM / PM
		: AM / PM
		: AM / PM
		: AM / PM
		: AM / PM
		: AM / PM
		: AM / PM
		: AM / PM
		: AM / PM
		: AM / PM
		: AM / PM
		: AM / PM

SIDE EFFECTS

ADDITIONAL NOTES

PHYSICAL CONDITION

SLEEP		WATER	
ENERGY		ACTIVITY	

📅 DATE		#️⃣ WEEK

💊 NAME	🌱 DOSAGE	⏱️ TIME
		: AM /
		: AM /
		: AM /
		: AM /
		: AM /
		: AM /
		: AM /
		: AM /
		: AM /
		: AM /
		: AM /
		: AM /
		: AM /
		: AM /
		: AM /

🤕 SIDE EFFECTS	📝 ADDITIONAL NOTES
•	
•	
•	
•	
•	

PHYSICAL CONDITION	
🌙 SLEEP	🥤 WATER
☀️ ENERGY	🏃 ACTIVITY

| 📅 DATE | | #️⃣ WEEK | |

🪴 NAME	🪴 DOSAGE	💊 TIME	
		:	AM / PM
		:	AM / PM
		:	AM / PM
		:	AM / PM
		:	AM / PM
		:	AM / PM
		:	AM / PM
		:	AM / PM
		:	AM / PM
		:	AM / PM
		:	AM / PM
		:	AM / PM
		:	AM / PM
		:	AM / PM
		:	AM / PM

🦠 SIDE EFFECTS	📝 ADDITIONAL NOTES

PHYSICAL CONDITION	
💤 SLEEP	🥛 WATER
🔋 ENERGY	🏃 ACTIVITY

📅 DATE		#️ WEEK	

💊 NAME	🌱 DOSAGE	⏰ TIME	
		:	AM / P
		:	AM / P
		:	AM / P
		:	AM / P
		:	AM / P
		:	AM / P
		:	AM / P
		:	AM / P
		:	AM / P
		:	AM / P
		:	AM / P
		:	AM / P
		:	AM / P
		:	AM / P
		:	AM / P

🧠 SIDE EFFECTS	📝 ADDITIONAL NOTES
·	
·	
·	
·	
·	

PHYSICAL CONDITION	
🌙 SLEEP	🥛 WATER
⚡ ENERGY	🏃 ACTIVITY

DATE	# WEEK

NAME	🌱 DOSAGE	⏰ TIME	
		:	AM / PM
		:	AM / PM
		:	AM / PM
		:	AM / PM
		:	AM / PM
		:	AM / PM
		:	AM / PM
		:	AM / PM
		:	AM / PM
		:	AM / PM
		:	AM / PM
		:	AM / PM
		:	AM / PM
		:	AM / PM
		:	AM / PM

SIDE EFFECTS	📝 ADDITIONAL NOTES

PHYSICAL CONDITION	
SLEEP	WATER
ENERGY	ACTIVITY

🔲 DATE		#️⃣ WEEK

💊 NAME	🌱 DOSAGE	⏱️ TIME
		: AM
		: AM
		: AM
		: AM
		: AM
		: AM
		: AM
		: AM
		: AM
		: AM
		: AM
		: AM
		: AM
		: AM
		: AM

🤕 SIDE EFFECTS	📝 ADDITIONAL NOTES
·	
·	
·	
·	
·	

PHYSICAL CONDITION	
🌙 SLEEP	🥤 WATER
⚡ ENERGY	🏃 ACTIVITY

DATE		# WEEK

NAME	DOSAGE	TIME
		: ____ AM / PM
		: ____ AM / PM
		: ____ AM / PM
		: ____ AM / PM
		: ____ AM / PM
		: ____ AM / PM
		: ____ AM / PM
		: ____ AM / PM
		: ____ AM / PM
		: ____ AM / PM
		: ____ AM / PM
		: ____ AM / PM
		: ____ AM / PM
		: ____ AM / PM
		: ____ AM / PM

SIDE EFFECTS

ADDITIONAL NOTES

PHYSICAL CONDITION

SLEEP		WATER	
ENERGY		ACTIVITY	

📅 DATE		# WEEK	

💊 NAME	🌱 DOSAGE	🍩 TIME	
		:	AM / P
		:	AM / P
		:	AM / P
		:	AM / P
		:	AM / P
		:	AM / P
		:	AM / P
		:	AM / P
		:	AM / P
		:	AM / P
		:	AM / P
		:	AM / P
		:	AM / P
		:	AM / P
		:	AM / P

🤕 SIDE EFFECTS	📝 ADDITIONAL NOTES
•	
•	
•	
•	
•	

PHYSICAL CONDITION	
🌙 SLEEP	🥛 WATER
☀️ ENERGY	🏃 ACTIVITY

📅 DATE		#️⃣ WEEK

🏷️ NAME	🌱 DOSAGE	💊 TIME
		: AM / PM
		: AM / PM
		: AM / PM
		: AM / PM
		: AM / PM
		: AM / PM
		: AM / PM
		: AM / PM
		: AM / PM
		: AM / PM
		: AM / PM
		: AM / PM
		: AM / PM
		: AM / PM
		: AM / PM
		: AM / PM

🦠 SIDE EFFECTS	📝 ADDITIONAL NOTES

PHYSICAL CONDITION	
✨ SLEEP ⬭⬭⬭⬭⬭	🥤 WATER ⬭⬭⬭⬭⬭
⚡ ENERGY ⬭⬭⬭⬭⬭	🏃 ACTIVITY ⬭⬭⬭⬭⬭

📅 DATE		#️⃣ WEEK

💊 NAME	🌿 DOSAGE	🕐 TIME
		: AM / P
		: AM / P
		: AM / P
		: AM / P
		: AM / P
		: AM / P
		: AM / P
		: AM / P
		: AM / P
		: AM / P
		: AM / P
		: AM / P
		: AM / P
		: AM / P
		: AM / P

🧠 SIDE EFFECTS	📝 ADDITIONAL NOTES
•	
•	
•	
•	
•	

PHYSICAL CONDITION		
🌙 SLEEP	💧 WATER	
⚡ ENERGY	🏃 ACTIVITY	

DATE		## WEEK

NAME	DOSAGE	TIME
		: AM / PM
		: AM / PM
		: AM / PM
		: AM / PM
		: AM / PM
		: AM / PM
		: AM / PM
		: AM / PM
		: AM / PM
		: AM / PM
		: AM / PM
		: AM / PM
		: AM / PM
		: AM / PM
		: AM / PM
		: AM / PM

SIDE EFFECTS	ADDITIONAL NOTES

PHYSICAL CONDITION

SLEEP		WATER	
ENERGY		ACTIVITY	

📅 DATE		# WEEK	

💊 NAME	🌱 DOSAGE	⏰ TIME	
		:	AM
		:	AM
		:	AM
		:	AM
		:	AM
		:	AM
		:	AM
		:	AM
		:	AM
		:	AM
		:	AM
		:	AM
		:	AM
		:	AM
		:	AM

🧠 SIDE EFFECTS	📝 ADDITIONAL NOTES
·	
·	
·	
·	
·	

PHYSICAL CONDITION	
🌙 SLEEP	🥛 WATER
⚡ ENERGY	🏃 ACTIVITY

DATE		# WEEK

NAME	DOSAGE	TIME
		: AM / PM
		: AM / PM
		: AM / PM
		: AM / PM
		: AM / PM
		: AM / PM
		: AM / PM
		: AM / PM
		: AM / PM
		: AM / PM
		: AM / PM
		: AM / PM
		: AM / PM
		: AM / PM
		: AM / PM

SIDE EFFECTS	ADDITIONAL NOTES

PHYSICAL CONDITION

SLEEP		WATER	
ENERGY		ACTIVITY	

📅 DATE		# WEEK	

💊 NAME	🌱 DOSAGE	⏰ TIME	
		:	AM / P
		:	AM / P
		:	AM / P
		:	AM / P
		:	AM / P
		:	AM / P
		:	AM / P
		:	AM / P
		:	AM / P
		:	AM / P
		:	AM / P
		:	AM / P
		:	AM / P
		:	AM / P
		:	AM / P

🧠 SIDE EFFECTS	📝 ADDITIONAL NOTES
•	
•	
•	
•	
•	

PHYSICAL CONDITION			
🌙 SLEEP	▭▭▭▭▭	🥛 WATER	▭▭▭▭▭
⚡ ENERGY	▭▭▭▭▭	🏃 ACTIVITY	▭▭▭▭▭

📓 DATE	# WEEK

🖊 NAME	🌱 DOSAGE	💊 TIME
		: _____ AM / PM
		: _____ AM / PM
		: _____ AM / PM
		: _____ AM / PM
		: _____ AM / PM
		: _____ AM / PM
		: _____ AM / PM
		: _____ AM / PM
		: _____ AM / PM
		: _____ AM / PM
		: _____ AM / PM
		: _____ AM / PM
		: _____ AM / PM
		: _____ AM / PM

🍷 SIDE EFFECTS	📝 ADDITIONAL NOTES

PHYSICAL CONDITION

💤 SLEEP	▭▭▭▭	🥛 WATER	▭▭▭▭
⚡ ENERGY	▭▭▭▭	🏃 ACTIVITY	▭▭▭▭

🗓 DATE		# WEEK

💊 NAME	🌱 DOSAGE	🕐 TIME
		: AM / P
		: AM / P
		: AM / P
		: AM / P
		: AM / P
		: AM / P
		: AM / P
		: AM / P
		: AM / P
		: AM / P
		: AM / P
		: AM / P
		: AM / P
		: AM / P
		: AM / P

🧠 SIDE EFFECTS	📝 ADDITIONAL NOTES
•	
•	
•	
•	
•	

PHYSICAL CONDITION	
🌙 SLEEP	💧 WATER
⚡ ENERGY	🏃 ACTIVITY

DATE		☐ WEEK

NAME	🌱 DOSAGE	🍥 TIME
		: AM / PM
		: AM / PM
		: AM / PM
		: AM / PM
		: AM / PM
		: AM / PM
		: AM / PM
		: AM / PM
		: AM / PM
		: AM / PM
		: AM / PM
		: AM / PM
		: AM / PM
		: AM / PM
		: AM / PM

SIDE EFFECTS	📝 ADDITIONAL NOTES

PHYSICAL CONDITION

SLEEP	▭▭▭▭▭	🥛 WATER	▭▭▭▭▭
ENERGY	▭▭▭▭▭	🏃 ACTIVITY	▭▭▭▭▭

📅 DATE		#️⃣ WEEK

💊 NAME	🌱 DOSAGE	⏰ TIME	
		:	AM
		:	AM
		:	AM
		:	AM
		:	AM
		:	AM
		:	AM
		:	AM
		:	AM
		:	AM
		:	AM
		:	AM
		:	AM
		:	AM
		:	AM

🗯 SIDE EFFECTS	📝 ADDITIONAL NOTES
•	
•	
•	
•	
•	

PHYSICAL CONDITION	
🌙 SLEEP	🥛 WATER
⚡ ENERGY	🏃 ACTIVITY

DATE	# WEEK

NAME	🌱 DOSAGE	⏰ TIME
		: AM / PM
		: AM / PM
		: AM / PM
		: AM / PM
		: AM / PM
		: AM / PM
		: AM / PM
		: AM / PM
		: AM / PM
		: AM / PM
		: AM / PM
		: AM / PM
		: AM / PM
		: AM / PM
		: AM / PM
		: AM / PM

SIDE EFFECTS	📝 ADDITIONAL NOTES

PHYSICAL CONDITION

SLEEP	⬜⬜⬜⬜⬜	WATER	⬜⬜⬜⬜⬜
ENERGY	⬜⬜⬜⬜⬜	ACTIVITY	⬜⬜⬜⬜⬜

📅 DATE		#️⃣ WEEK	

💊 NAME	🪴 DOSAGE	⏲️ TIME	
		:	AM /
		:	AM /
		:	AM /
		:	AM /
		:	AM /
		:	AM /
		:	AM /
		:	AM /
		:	AM /
		:	AM /
		:	AM /
		:	AM /
		:	AM /
		:	AM /
		:	AM /

🗣️ SIDE EFFECTS	📝 ADDITIONAL NOTES
•	
•	
•	
•	
•	

PHYSICAL CONDITION	
🌙 SLEEP	🥛 WATER
🔆 ENERGY	🏃 ACTIVITY

📅 DATE		# WEEK

✏️ NAME	🪴 DOSAGE	⏰ TIME
		: AM / PM
		: AM / PM
		: AM / PM
		: AM / PM
		: AM / PM
		: AM / PM
		: AM / PM
		: AM / PM
		: AM / PM
		: AM / PM
		: AM / PM
		: AM / PM
		: AM / PM
		: AM / PM
		: AM / PM

📝 SIDE EFFECTS

📝 ADDITIONAL NOTES

PHYSICAL CONDITION

SLEEP		WATER	
ENERGY		ACTIVITY	

📅 DATE				# WEEK		

💊 NAME	🌱 DOSAGE	🕐 TIME	
		:	AM / P
		:	AM / P
		:	AM / P
		:	AM / P
		:	AM / P
		:	AM / P
		:	AM / P
		:	AM / P
		:	AM / P
		:	AM / P
		:	AM / P
		:	AM / P
		:	AM / P
		:	AM / P
		:	AM / P

🧠 SIDE EFFECTS	📝 ADDITIONAL NOTES
•	
•	
•	
•	
•	

PHYSICAL CONDITION

🌙 SLEEP		🥛 WATER	
🔋 ENERGY		🏃 ACTIVITY	

DATE	# WEEK

NAME	🌱 DOSAGE	💊 TIME
		: AM / PM
		: AM / PM
		: AM / PM
		: AM / PM
		: AM / PM
		: AM / PM
		: AM / PM
		: AM / PM
		: AM / PM
		: AM / PM
		: AM / PM
		: AM / PM
		: AM / PM
		: AM / PM
		: AM / PM

SIDE EFFECTS	📝 ADDITIONAL NOTES

PHYSICAL CONDITION

SLEEP		WATER	
ENERGY		🏃 ACTIVITY	

📅 DATE		# WEEK

💊 NAME	🌱 DOSAGE	🕙 TIME
		: AM
		: AM
		: AM
		: AM
		: AM
		: AM
		: AM
		: AM
		: AM
		: AM
		: AM
		: AM
		: AM
		: AM
		: AM

🤕 SIDE EFFECTS	📝 ADDITIONAL NOTES
.	
.	
.	
.	
.	

PHYSICAL CONDITION	
🌙 SLEEP	💧 WATER
⚡ ENERGY	🏃 ACTIVITY

DATE	# WEEK

NAME	DOSAGE	TIME
		: ____ AM / PM
		: ____ AM / PM
		: ____ AM / PM
		: ____ AM / PM
		: ____ AM / PM
		: ____ AM / PM
		: ____ AM / PM
		: ____ AM / PM
		: ____ AM / PM
		: ____ AM / PM
		: ____ AM / PM
		: ____ AM / PM
		: ____ AM / PM
		: ____ AM / PM
		: ____ AM / PM

SIDE EFFECTS	ADDITIONAL NOTES

PHYSICAL CONDITION

SLEEP		WATER	
ENERGY		ACTIVITY	

📅 DATE		#️⃣ WEEK

💊 NAME	🌱 DOSAGE	🕐 TIME	
		:	AM /
		:	AM /
		:	AM /
		:	AM /
		:	AM /
		:	AM /
		:	AM /
		:	AM /
		:	AM /
		:	AM /
		:	AM /
		:	AM /
		:	AM /
		:	AM /
		:	AM /

🧠 SIDE EFFECTS	📝 ADDITIONAL NOTES
•	
•	
•	
•	
•	

PHYSICAL CONDITION			
🌙 SLEEP	▭▭▭▭▭	🥛 WATER	▭▭▭▭▭
⚡ ENERGY	▭▭▭▭▭	🏃 ACTIVITY	▭▭▭▭▭

📅 DATE		# WEEK

✍ NAME	🌿 DOSAGE	🕐 TIME
		: AM / PM
		: AM / PM
		: AM / PM
		: AM / PM
		: AM / PM
		: AM / PM
		: AM / PM
		: AM / PM
		: AM / PM
		: AM / PM
		: AM / PM
		: AM / PM
		: AM / PM
		: AM / PM
		: AM / PM
		: AM / PM

🧴 SIDE EFFECTS	📝 ADDITIONAL NOTES

PHYSICAL CONDITION

😴 SLEEP	▭▭▭▭▭	🥛 WATER	▭▭▭▭▭
⚡ ENERGY	▭▭▭▭▭	🏃 ACTIVITY	▭▭▭▭▭

📅 DATE		# WEEK	

⊘ NAME	🌱 DOSAGE	🕐 TIME	
		:	AM / P
		:	AM / P
		:	AM / P
		:	AM / P
		:	AM / P
		:	AM / P
		:	AM / P
		:	AM / P
		:	AM / P
		:	AM / P
		:	AM / P
		:	AM / P
		:	AM / P
		:	AM / P
		:	AM / P

🗣 SIDE EFFECTS	📝 ADDITIONAL NOTES
•	
•	
•	
•	
•	

PHYSICAL CONDITION

🌙 SLEEP		🥛 WATER	
🔋 ENERGY		🏃 ACTIVITY	

DATE		# WEEK

NAME	💊 DOSAGE	💊 TIME
		: AM / PM
		: AM / PM
		: AM / PM
		: AM / PM
		: AM / PM
		: AM / PM
		: AM / PM
		: AM / PM
		: AM / PM
		: AM / PM
		: AM / PM
		: AM / PM
		: AM / PM
		: AM / PM
		: AM / PM
		: AM / PM

SIDE EFFECTS	📝 ADDITIONAL NOTES

PHYSICAL CONDITION	
SLEEP ▭▭▭▭▭	🥛 WATER ▭▭▭▭▭
ENERGY ▭▭▭▭▭	🏃 ACTIVITY ▭▭▭▭▭

📅 DATE		#️⃣ WEEK

💊 NAME	🌱 DOSAGE	🕐 TIME
		: AM
		: AM
		: AM
		: AM
		: AM
		: AM
		: AM
		: AM
		: AM
		: AM
		: AM
		: AM
		: AM
		: AM
		: AM

🧠 SIDE EFFECTS	📝 ADDITIONAL NOTES
•	
•	
•	
•	
•	

PHYSICAL CONDITION	
🌙 SLEEP	🥤 WATER
⚡ ENERGY	🏃 ACTIVITY

DATE		# WEEK	

NAME	DOSAGE	TIME	
		:	AM / PM
		:	AM / PM
		:	AM / PM
		:	AM / PM
		:	AM / PM
		:	AM / PM
		:	AM / PM
		:	AM / PM
		:	AM / PM
		:	AM / PM
		:	AM / PM
		:	AM / PM
		:	AM / PM
		:	AM / PM
		:	AM / PM

SIDE EFFECTS	ADDITIONAL NOTES

PHYSICAL CONDITION

SLEEP		WATER	
ENERGY		ACTIVITY	

📅 DATE			#️⃣ WEEK

💊 NAME	🌱 DOSAGE	🕐 TIME	
		:	AM /
		:	AM /
		:	AM /
		:	AM /
		:	AM /
		:	AM /
		:	AM /
		:	AM /
		:	AM /
		:	AM /
		:	AM /
		:	AM /
		:	AM /
		:	AM /
		:	AM /

🧠 SIDE EFFECTS	📝 ADDITIONAL NOTES
•	
•	
•	
•	
•	

PHYSICAL CONDITION	
🌙 SLEEP	🥤 WATER
🔆 ENERGY	🏃 ACTIVITY

📓 DATE		🔢 WEEK

🖊 NAME	🪴 DOSAGE	🕑 TIME
		: AM / PM
		: AM / PM
		: AM / PM
		: AM / PM
		: AM / PM
		: AM / PM
		: AM / PM
		: AM / PM
		: AM / PM
		: AM / PM
		: AM / PM
		: AM / PM
		: AM / PM
		: AM / PM
		: AM / PM
		: AM / PM

🧪 SIDE EFFECTS	📝 ADDITIONAL NOTES

PHYSICAL CONDITION

SLEEP		WATER	
⚡ ENERGY		🏃 ACTIVITY	

📅 DATE		# WEEK

💊 NAME	🧪 DOSAGE	⏰ TIME
		: AM / P
		: AM / P
		: AM / P
		: AM / P
		: AM / P
		: AM / P
		: AM / P
		: AM / P
		: AM / P
		: AM / P
		: AM / P
		: AM / P
		: AM / P
		: AM / P
		: AM / P

🧠 SIDE EFFECTS	📝 ADDITIONAL NOTES
•	
•	
•	
•	
•	

PHYSICAL CONDITION

🌙 SLEEP		🥤 WATER	
⚡ ENERGY		🏃 ACTIVITY	

DATE	# WEEK

NAME	🌱 DOSAGE	⏰ TIME	
		:	AM / PM
		:	AM / PM
		:	AM / PM
		:	AM / PM
		:	AM / PM
		:	AM / PM
		:	AM / PM
		:	AM / PM
		:	AM / PM
		:	AM / PM
		:	AM / PM
		:	AM / PM
		:	AM / PM
		:	AM / PM
		:	AM / PM
		:	AM / PM

SIDE EFFECTS	📝 ADDITIONAL NOTES

PHYSICAL CONDITION	
SLEEP ▭▭▭▭▭	🥛 WATER ▭▭▭▭▭
ENERGY ▭▭▭▭▭	🏃 ACTIVITY ▭▭▭▭▭

📅 DATE		# WEEK

💊 NAME	🌱 DOSAGE	🕐 TIME
		: AM
		: AM
		: AM
		: AM
		: AM
		: AM
		: AM
		: AM
		: AM
		: AM
		: AM
		: AM
		: AM
		: AM
		: AM

🤕 SIDE EFFECTS	📝 ADDITIONAL NOTES
•	
•	
•	
•	
•	

PHYSICAL CONDITION	
🌙 SLEEP ▭▭▭▭▭	🥛 WATER ▭▭▭▭▭
⚡ ENERGY ▭▭▭▭▭	🏃 ACTIVITY ▭▭▭▭▭

DATE		# WEEK	

NAME	DOSAGE	TIME	
		:	AM / PM
		:	AM / PM
		:	AM / PM
		:	AM / PM
		:	AM / PM
		:	AM / PM
		:	AM / PM
		:	AM / PM
		:	AM / PM
		:	AM / PM
		:	AM / PM
		:	AM / PM
		:	AM / PM
		:	AM / PM
		:	AM / PM

SIDE EFFECTS	ADDITIONAL NOTES

PHYSICAL CONDITION

SLEEP		WATER	
ENERGY		ACTIVITY	

📅 DATE		# WEEK

💊 NAME	🌱 DOSAGE	🕐 TIME	
		:	AM /
		:	AM /
		:	AM /
		:	AM /
		:	AM /
		:	AM /
		:	AM /
		:	AM /
		:	AM /
		:	AM /
		:	AM /
		:	AM /
		:	AM /
		:	AM /
		:	AM /

🗣 SIDE EFFECTS	📝 ADDITIONAL NOTES
•	
•	
•	
•	
•	

PHYSICAL CONDITION	
🌙 SLEEP	🥤 WATER
🔆 ENERGY	🏃 ACTIVITY

📅 DATE		#️⃣ WEEK

🧪 NAME	🌱 DOSAGE	🍬 TIME
		: AM / PM
		: AM / PM
		: AM / PM
		: AM / PM
		: AM / PM
		: AM / PM
		: AM / PM
		: AM / PM
		: AM / PM
		: AM / PM
		: AM / PM
		: AM / PM
		: AM / PM
		: AM / PM
		: AM / PM

🦠 SIDE EFFECTS	📝 ADDITIONAL NOTES

PHYSICAL CONDITION		
💤 SLEEP		🥛 WATER
⚡ ENERGY		🏃 ACTIVITY

📅 DATE			# WEEK	

💊 NAME	🌿 DOSAGE	🕐 TIME	
		:	AM / PM
		:	AM / PM
		:	AM / PM
		:	AM / PM
		:	AM / PM
		:	AM / PM
		:	AM / PM
		:	AM / PM
		:	AM / PM
		:	AM / PM
		:	AM / PM
		:	AM / PM
		:	AM / PM
		:	AM / PM
		:	AM / PM

🧠 SIDE EFFECTS	📝 ADDITIONAL NOTES
•	
•	
•	
•	
•	

PHYSICAL CONDITION

🌙 SLEEP		🥛 WATER	
⚡ ENERGY		🏃 ACTIVITY	

DATE		# WEEK

NAME	🌱 DOSAGE	💊 TIME
		: AM / PM
		: AM / PM
		: AM / PM
		: AM / PM
		: AM / PM
		: AM / PM
		: AM / PM
		: AM / PM
		: AM / PM
		: AM / PM
		: AM / PM
		: AM / PM
		: AM / PM
		: AM / PM
		: AM / PM

SIDE EFFECTS	📝 ADDITIONAL NOTES

PHYSICAL CONDITION		
SLEEP	🥛 WATER	
ENERGY	🏃 ACTIVITY	

📅 DATE		# WEEK	

💊 NAME	🌱 DOSAGE	⏰ TIME	
		:	AM
		:	AM
		:	AM
		:	AM
		:	AM
		:	AM
		:	AM
		:	AM
		:	AM
		:	AM
		:	AM
		:	AM
		:	AM
		:	AM
		:	AM

🧠 SIDE EFFECTS	📝 ADDITIONAL NOTES
•	
•	
•	
•	
•	

PHYSICAL CONDITION	
🌙 SLEEP	💧 WATER
⚡ ENERGY	🏃 ACTIVITY

📅 DATE		# WEEK

💊 NAME	💊 DOSAGE	🕐 TIME	
		:	AM / PM
		:	AM / PM
		:	AM / PM
		:	AM / PM
		:	AM / PM
		:	AM / PM
		:	AM / PM
		:	AM / PM
		:	AM / PM
		:	AM / PM
		:	AM / PM
		:	AM / PM
		:	AM / PM
		:	AM / PM
		:	AM / PM

⚡ SIDE EFFECTS	📝 ADDITIONAL NOTES

PHYSICAL CONDITION

SLEEP	⬭⬭⬭⬭⬭	🥛 WATER	⬭⬭⬭⬭⬭
ENERGY	⬭⬭⬭⬭⬭	🏃 ACTIVITY	⬭⬭⬭⬭⬭

📅 DATE		#️⃣ WEEK	

💊 NAME	🌱 DOSAGE	🍽️ TIME	
		:	AM /
		:	AM /
		:	AM /
		:	AM /
		:	AM /
		:	AM /
		:	AM /
		:	AM /
		:	AM /
		:	AM /
		:	AM /
		:	AM /
		:	AM /
		:	AM /
		:	AM /

😷 SIDE EFFECTS	📝 ADDITIONAL NOTES
•	
•	
•	
•	
•	

PHYSICAL CONDITION		
🌙 SLEEP	💧 WATER	
☀️ ENERGY	🏃 ACTIVITY	

DATE		# WEEK

NAME	DOSAGE	TIME
		: AM / PM
		: AM / PM
		: AM / PM
		: AM / PM
		: AM / PM
		: AM / PM
		: AM / PM
		: AM / PM
		: AM / PM
		: AM / PM
		: AM / PM
		: AM / PM
		: AM / PM
		: AM / PM
		: AM / PM

SIDE EFFECTS	ADDITIONAL NOTES

PHYSICAL CONDITION	
SLEEP	WATER
ENERGY	ACTIVITY

📅 DATE		# WEEK

💊 NAME	💊 DOSAGE	⏰ TIME	
		:	AM / P
		:	AM / P
		:	AM / P
		:	AM / P
		:	AM / P
		:	AM / P
		:	AM / P
		:	AM / P
		:	AM / P
		:	AM / P
		:	AM / P
		:	AM / P
		:	AM / P
		:	AM / P
		:	AM / P

🗣 SIDE EFFECTS	📝 ADDITIONAL NOTES
•	
•	
•	
•	
•	

PHYSICAL CONDITION	
🌙 SLEEP	💧 WATER
⚡ ENERGY	🏃 ACTIVITY

DATE		# WEEK	

NAME	🌱 DOSAGE	⏰ TIME	
		:	AM / PM
		:	AM / PM
		:	AM / PM
		:	AM / PM
		:	AM / PM
		:	AM / PM
		:	AM / PM
		:	AM / PM
		:	AM / PM
		:	AM / PM
		:	AM / PM
		:	AM / PM
		:	AM / PM
		:	AM / PM
		:	AM / PM

SIDE EFFECTS	📝 ADDITIONAL NOTES

PHYSICAL CONDITION			
SLEEP		WATER	
ENERGY		🏃 ACTIVITY	

🗓 DATE		# WEEK	

💊 NAME	🌱 DOSAGE	⏰ TIME	
		:	AM
		:	AM
		:	AM
		:	AM
		:	AM
		:	AM
		:	AM
		:	AM
		:	AM
		:	AM
		:	AM
		:	AM
		:	AM
		:	AM
		:	AM

🧠 SIDE EFFECTS	📝 ADDITIONAL NOTES
•	
•	
•	
•	
•	

PHYSICAL CONDITION	
🌙 SLEEP	💧 WATER
⚡ ENERGY	🏃 ACTIVITY

DATE	# WEEK

NAME	DOSAGE	TIME
		: AM / PM
		: AM / PM
		: AM / PM
		: AM / PM
		: AM / PM
		: AM / PM
		: AM / PM
		: AM / PM
		: AM / PM
		: AM / PM
		: AM / PM
		: AM / PM
		: AM / PM
		: AM / PM
		: AM / PM

SIDE EFFECTS	ADDITIONAL NOTES

PHYSICAL CONDITION	
SLEEP	WATER
ENERGY	ACTIVITY

📅 DATE		#️⃣ WEEK

💊 NAME	🌱 DOSAGE	⏰ TIME	
		:	AM /
		:	AM /
		:	AM /
		:	AM /
		:	AM /
		:	AM /
		:	AM /
		:	AM /
		:	AM /
		:	AM /
		:	AM /
		:	AM /
		:	AM /
		:	AM /
		:	AM /

😷 SIDE EFFECTS	📝 ADDITIONAL NOTES
•	
•	
•	
•	
•	

PHYSICAL CONDITION	
🌙 SLEEP	🥛 WATER
⚡ ENERGY	🏃 ACTIVITY

📅 DATE		# WEEK

🔖 NAME	🌱 DOSAGE	💊 TIME
		: AM / PM
		: AM / PM
		: AM / PM
		: AM / PM
		: AM / PM
		: AM / PM
		: AM / PM
		: AM / PM
		: AM / PM
		: AM / PM
		: AM / PM
		: AM / PM
		: AM / PM
		: AM / PM
		: AM / PM

🦵 SIDE EFFECTS	📝 ADDITIONAL NOTES

PHYSICAL CONDITION	
💤 SLEEP ⬜⬜⬜⬜⬜	🥛 WATER ⬜⬜⬜⬜⬜
⚡ ENERGY ⬜⬜⬜⬜⬜	🏃 ACTIVITY ⬜⬜⬜⬜⬜

📅 DATE	# WEEK

💊 NAME	🌿 DOSAGE	⏰ TIME
		: AM / PM
		: AM / PM
		: AM / PM
		: AM / PM
		: AM / PM
		: AM / PM
		: AM / PM
		: AM / PM
		: AM / PM
		: AM / PM
		: AM / PM
		: AM / PM
		: AM / PM
		: AM / PM
		: AM / PM

🧠 SIDE EFFECTS	📝 ADDITIONAL NOTES
•	
•	
•	
•	
•	

PHYSICAL CONDITION	
🌙 SLEEP	💧 WATER
⚡ ENERGY	🏃 ACTIVITY

DATE	# WEEK

NAME	🪴 DOSAGE	⏰ TIME
		: AM / PM
		: AM / PM
		: AM / PM
		: AM / PM
		: AM / PM
		: AM / PM
		: AM / PM
		: AM / PM
		: AM / PM
		: AM / PM
		: AM / PM
		: AM / PM
		: AM / PM
		: AM / PM
		: AM / PM
		: AM / PM

SIDE EFFECTS	📝 ADDITIONAL NOTES

PHYSICAL CONDITION	
SLEEP	WATER
ENERGY	ACTIVITY

📅 DATE		# WEEK

💊 NAME	🌿 DOSAGE	🕐 TIME
		: AM
		: AM
		: AM
		: AM
		: AM
		: AM
		: AM
		: AM
		: AM
		: AM
		: AM
		: AM
		: AM
		: AM
		: AM

🧠 SIDE EFFECTS	📝 ADDITIONAL NOTES
•	
•	
•	
•	
•	

PHYSICAL CONDITION	
🌙 SLEEP	💧 WATER
⚡ ENERGY	🏃 ACTIVITY

DATE		# WEEK

NAME	DOSAGE	TIME
		: AM / PM
		: AM / PM
		: AM / PM
		: AM / PM
		: AM / PM
		: AM / PM
		: AM / PM
		: AM / PM
		: AM / PM
		: AM / PM
		: AM / PM
		: AM / PM
		: AM / PM
		: AM / PM
		: AM / PM
		: AM / PM

SIDE EFFECTS

ADDITIONAL NOTES

PHYSICAL CONDITION

SLEEP		WATER	
ENERGY		ACTIVITY	

📅 DATE		# WEEK

💊 NAME	🌱 DOSAGE	⏱ TIME	
		:	AM /
		:	AM /
		:	AM /
		:	AM /
		:	AM /
		:	AM /
		:	AM /
		:	AM /
		:	AM /
		:	AM /
		:	AM /
		:	AM /
		:	AM /
		:	AM /
		:	AM /

😵 SIDE EFFECTS	📝 ADDITIONAL NOTES
•	
•	
•	
•	
•	

PHYSICAL CONDITION		
🌙 SLEEP	💧 WATER	
⚡ ENERGY	🏃 ACTIVITY	

📅 DATE		# WEEK

🔖 NAME	🌱 DOSAGE	🍬 TIME
		:　　　　AM / PM
		:　　　　AM / PM
		:　　　　AM / PM
		:　　　　AM / PM
		:　　　　AM / PM
		:　　　　AM / PM
		:　　　　AM / PM
		:　　　　AM / PM
		:　　　　AM / PM
		:　　　　AM / PM
		:　　　　AM / PM
		:　　　　AM / PM
		:　　　　AM / PM
		:　　　　AM / PM
		:　　　　AM / PM

🌿 SIDE EFFECTS	📝 ADDITIONAL NOTES

PHYSICAL CONDITION	
💤 SLEEP	🥤 WATER
⚡ ENERGY	🏃 ACTIVITY

📅 DATE		# WEEK

💊 NAME	🌱 DOSAGE	🕑 TIME	
		:	AM / P
		:	AM / P
		:	AM / P
		:	AM / P
		:	AM / P
		:	AM / P
		:	AM / P
		:	AM / P
		:	AM / P
		:	AM / P
		:	AM / P
		:	AM / P
		:	AM / P
		:	AM / P
		:	AM / P

🧠 SIDE EFFECTS	📝 ADDITIONAL NOTES
•	
•	
•	
•	
•	

PHYSICAL CONDITION

🌙 SLEEP		🥛 WATER	
⚡ ENERGY		🏃 ACTIVITY	

DATE		# WEEK

NAME	🌱 DOSAGE	💊 TIME
		: AM / PM
		: AM / PM
		: AM / PM
		: AM / PM
		: AM / PM
		: AM / PM
		: AM / PM
		: AM / PM
		: AM / PM
		: AM / PM
		: AM / PM
		: AM / PM
		: AM / PM
		: AM / PM
		: AM / PM

SIDE EFFECTS	📝 ADDITIONAL NOTES

PHYSICAL CONDITION	
SLEEP	🥛 WATER
ENERGY	🏃 ACTIVITY

🗓 DATE		# WEEK

💊 NAME	🌱 DOSAGE	⏰ TIME	
		:	AM
		:	AM
		:	AM
		:	AM
		:	AM
		:	AM
		:	AM
		:	AM
		:	AM
		:	AM
		:	AM
		:	AM
		:	AM
		:	AM
		:	AM

🤕 SIDE EFFECTS	📝 ADDITIONAL NOTES
•	
•	
•	
•	
•	

PHYSICAL CONDITION	
🌙 SLEEP	💧 WATER
⚡ ENERGY	🏃 ACTIVITY

DATE			# WEEK	

⌀ NAME	🌱 DOSAGE	🕘 TIME	
		:	AM / PM
		:	AM / PM
		:	AM / PM
		:	AM / PM
		:	AM / PM
		:	AM / PM
		:	AM / PM
		:	AM / PM
		:	AM / PM
		:	AM / PM
		:	AM / PM
		:	AM / PM
		:	AM / PM
		:	AM / PM
		:	AM / PM

⅄ SIDE EFFECTS	🖉 ADDITIONAL NOTES

PHYSICAL CONDITION	
☀ SLEEP	🧊 WATER
⚡ ENERGY	🏃 ACTIVITY

📅 DATE		# WEEK

💊 NAME	🌱 DOSAGE	⏲ TIME
		: AM /
		: AM /
		: AM /
		: AM /
		: AM /
		: AM /
		: AM /
		: AM /
		: AM /
		: AM /
		: AM /
		: AM /
		: AM /
		: AM /
		: AM /

🤕 SIDE EFFECTS	📝 ADDITIONAL NOTES
•	
•	
•	
•	
•	

PHYSICAL CONDITION		
🌙 SLEEP		🥤 WATER
⚡ ENERGY		🏃 ACTIVITY

📓 DATE		# WEEK

🗒 NAME	🪴 DOSAGE	🍬 TIME
		: AM / PM
		: AM / PM
		: AM / PM
		: AM / PM
		: AM / PM
		: AM / PM
		: AM / PM
		: AM / PM
		: AM / PM
		: AM / PM
		: AM / PM
		: AM / PM
		: AM / PM
		: AM / PM
		: AM / PM

🧫 SIDE EFFECTS	📝 ADDITIONAL NOTES

PHYSICAL CONDITION	
SLEEP	WATER
ENERGY	ACTIVITY

📅 DATE		# WEEK

💊 NAME	🌱 DOSAGE	🕐 TIME
		: AM / PM
		: AM / PM
		: AM / PM
		: AM / PM
		: AM / PM
		: AM / PM
		: AM / PM
		: AM / PM
		: AM / PM
		: AM / PM
		: AM / PM
		: AM / PM
		: AM / PM
		: AM / PM
		: AM / PM

🧠 SIDE EFFECTS	📝 ADDITIONAL NOTES
•	
•	
•	
•	
•	

PHYSICAL CONDITION			
🌙 SLEEP		🥛 WATER	
⚡ ENERGY		🏃 ACTIVITY	

DATE		# WEEK

NAME	🌱 DOSAGE	🕐 TIME	
		:	AM / PM
		:	AM / PM
		:	AM / PM
		:	AM / PM
		:	AM / PM
		:	AM / PM
		:	AM / PM
		:	AM / PM
		:	AM / PM
		:	AM / PM
		:	AM / PM
		:	AM / PM
		:	AM / PM
		:	AM / PM
		:	AM / PM
		:	AM / PM

SIDE EFFECTS	📝 ADDITIONAL NOTES

PHYSICAL CONDITION		
SLEEP	WATER	
ENERGY	ACTIVITY	

📅 DATE		# WEEK	

💊 NAME	🌿 DOSAGE	🕐 TIME	
		:	AM
		:	AM
		:	AM
		:	AM
		:	AM
		:	AM
		:	AM
		:	AM
		:	AM
		:	AM
		:	AM
		:	AM
		:	AM
		:	AM
		:	AM

🤕 SIDE EFFECTS	📝 ADDITIONAL NOTES
·	
·	
·	
·	
·	

PHYSICAL CONDITION	
🌙 SLEEP	💧 WATER
⚡ ENERGY	🏃 ACTIVITY

📓 DATE			🗓️ WEEK	

🖊️ NAME	🌱 DOSAGE	⏰ TIME	
		:	AM / PM
		:	AM / PM
		:	AM / PM
		:	AM / PM
		:	AM / PM
		:	AM / PM
		:	AM / PM
		:	AM / PM
		:	AM / PM
		:	AM / PM
		:	AM / PM
		:	AM / PM
		:	AM / PM
		:	AM / PM
		:	AM / PM

🧴 SIDE EFFECTS	📝 ADDITIONAL NOTES

PHYSICAL CONDITION	
🌙 SLEEP	🥤 WATER
⚡ ENERGY	🏃 ACTIVITY

🗓 DATE		#️⃣ WEEK

💊 NAME	🌱 DOSAGE	⏰ TIME
		: AM /
		: AM /
		: AM /
		: AM /
		: AM /
		: AM /
		: AM /
		: AM /
		: AM /
		: AM /
		: AM /
		: AM /
		: AM /
		: AM /
		: AM /

🧠 SIDE EFFECTS	📝 ADDITIONAL NOTES
•	
•	
•	
•	
•	

PHYSICAL CONDITION

🌙 SLEEP	⬚⬚⬚⬚⬚	🥛 WATER	⬚⬚⬚⬚⬚
⚡ ENERGY	⬚⬚⬚⬚⬚	🏃 ACTIVITY	⬚⬚⬚⬚⬚

📅 DATE		# WEEK	

⚗️ NAME	💊 DOSAGE	🕐 TIME	
		:	AM / PM
		:	AM / PM
		:	AM / PM
		:	AM / PM
		:	AM / PM
		:	AM / PM
		:	AM / PM
		:	AM / PM
		:	AM / PM
		:	AM / PM
		:	AM / PM
		:	AM / PM
		:	AM / PM
		:	AM / PM
		:	AM / PM

🦠 SIDE EFFECTS	📝 ADDITIONAL NOTES

PHYSICAL CONDITION	
💤 SLEEP	🥛 WATER
⚡ ENERGY	🏃 ACTIVITY

📅 DATE		# WEEK

💊 NAME	🌱 DOSAGE	⏰ TIME
		: AM / P
		: AM / P
		: AM / P
		: AM / P
		: AM / P
		: AM / P
		: AM / P
		: AM / P
		: AM / P
		: AM / P
		: AM / P
		: AM / P
		: AM / P
		: AM / P
		: AM / P

🗣 SIDE EFFECTS	📝 ADDITIONAL NOTES
•	
•	
•	
•	
•	

PHYSICAL CONDITION	
🌙 SLEEP	🥛 WATER
⚡ ENERGY	🏃 ACTIVITY

DATE	# WEEK

NAME	🪴 DOSAGE	🕑 TIME
		: AM / PM
		: AM / PM
		: AM / PM
		: AM / PM
		: AM / PM
		: AM / PM
		: AM / PM
		: AM / PM
		: AM / PM
		: AM / PM
		: AM / PM
		: AM / PM
		: AM / PM
		: AM / PM
		: AM / PM

SIDE EFFECTS	📝 ADDITIONAL NOTES

PHYSICAL CONDITION		
SLEEP	🥛 WATER	
ENERGY	🏃 ACTIVITY	

📅 DATE		# WEEK

💊 NAME	🌱 DOSAGE	⏰ TIME
		: ___ AM
		: ___ AM
		: ___ AM
		: ___ AM
		: ___ AM
		: ___ AM
		: ___ AM
		: ___ AM
		: ___ AM
		: ___ AM
		: ___ AM
		: ___ AM
		: ___ AM
		: ___ AM
		: ___ AM

🤕 SIDE EFFECTS	📝 ADDITIONAL NOTES
•	
•	
•	
•	
•	

PHYSICAL CONDITION	
🌙 SLEEP	🥤 WATER
⚡ ENERGY	🏃 ACTIVITY

📋 DATE		# WEEK

🌿 NAME	💊 DOSAGE	🕐 TIME
		: AM / PM
		: AM / PM
		: AM / PM
		: AM / PM
		: AM / PM
		: AM / PM
		: AM / PM
		: AM / PM
		: AM / PM
		: AM / PM
		: AM / PM
		: AM / PM
		: AM / PM
		: AM / PM
		: AM / PM

🦴 SIDE EFFECTS	📝 ADDITIONAL NOTES

PHYSICAL CONDITION

☀ SLEEP	⬜⬜⬜⬜⬜	🥛 WATER	⬜⬜⬜⬜⬜
⚡ ENERGY	⬜⬜⬜⬜⬜	🏃 ACTIVITY	⬜⬜⬜⬜⬜

📅 DATE		# WEEK	

💊 NAME	🌱 DOSAGE	🕐 TIME	
		:	AM /
		:	AM /
		:	AM /
		:	AM /
		:	AM /
		:	AM /
		:	AM /
		:	AM /
		:	AM /
		:	AM /
		:	AM /
		:	AM /
		:	AM /
		:	AM /
		:	AM /

🧠 SIDE EFFECTS	📝 ADDITIONAL NOTES
·	
·	
·	
·	
·	

PHYSICAL CONDITION	
🌙 SLEEP	🥛 WATER
☀️ ENERGY	🏃 ACTIVITY

🖊 DATE		# WEEK

✏️ NAME	🌱 DOSAGE	💊 TIME
		: AM / PM
		: AM / PM
		: AM / PM
		: AM / PM
		: AM / PM
		: AM / PM
		: AM / PM
		: AM / PM
		: AM / PM
		: AM / PM
		: AM / PM
		: AM / PM
		: AM / PM
		: AM / PM
		: AM / PM

🦠 SIDE EFFECTS	📝 ADDITIONAL NOTES

PHYSICAL CONDITION	
💤 SLEEP	🥛 WATER
⚡ ENERGY	🏃 ACTIVITY

📅 DATE		#️⃣ WEEK

💊 NAME	🌱 DOSAGE	⏰ TIME
		: AM / P
		: AM / P
		: AM / P
		: AM / P
		: AM / P
		: AM / P
		: AM / P
		: AM / P
		: AM / P
		: AM / P
		: AM / P
		: AM / P
		: AM / P
		: AM / P
		: AM / P

🧠 SIDE EFFECTS	📝 ADDITIONAL NOTES
·	
·	
·	
·	
·	

PHYSICAL CONDITION

🌙 SLEEP		🥤 WATER	
⚡ ENERGY		🏃 ACTIVITY	

Made in the USA
Las Vegas, NV
28 January 2024

85020725R00059